DR. BARBARA CURE FOR DIABETES

The Comprehensive Guide to Treating and Curing Diabetes with Barbara O'Neill's Recommended Natural Foods

Billy Arthur

Table of Contents

Chapter 1
Introduction to Dr. Barbara and Her Healing Philosophy

Dr. Barbara stands as a beacon of innovation in the realm of holistic health and natural medicine, particularly in the field of diabetes management. With a wealth of experience in naturopathic medicine and a deep-rooted commitment to empowering individuals on their health journey, Dr. Barbara has become a trusted authority in alternative therapies. At the heart of her practice lies a profound philosophy that emphasizes treating the root cause of ailments, fostering holistic wellness, and harnessing the body's innate healing abilities.

Dr. Barbara's journey into holistic health began with a fervent desire to explore alternative approaches to traditional medicine. Drawing inspiration from diverse healing modalities and ancient wisdom traditions, she embarked on a quest to uncover natural remedies and lifestyle interventions that promote optimal health and vitality. Through years of dedicated research, clinical practice, and ongoing education, Dr. Barbara has refined her approach to healing, blending the best of traditional wisdom with modern science to offer comprehensive and personalized care to her patients.

Central to Dr. Barbara's healing philosophy is the belief that true health encompasses more than just the absence of disease—it encompasses harmony and balance in all aspects of life. She recognizes the interconnectedness of the body, mind, and spirit, understanding that imbalances in one area can manifest as symptoms in another. With this holistic perspective, Dr. Barbara seeks to address the underlying causes of illness, rather than merely managing symptoms, empowering individuals to take an active role in their health and well-being.

In the realm of diabetes management, Dr. Barbara's approach is no less revolutionary. Recognizing the limitations of conventional treatments and the need for a more integrative approach, she advocates for a holistic approach that addresses diet, lifestyle, supplementation, and mind-body practices. By emphasizing the importance of nutrition, herbal remedies, exercise, stress management, and self-care, Dr. Barbara equips individuals with the tools they need to thrive in their journey towards optimal health and vitality.

As we embark on this exploration of Dr. Barbara's healing philosophy, we invite you to delve deeper into the principles and practices that underpin her approach to wellness. By embracing a holistic perspective and tapping into the body's natural healing abilities, Dr. Barbara offers hope and empowerment to all those seeking a path to vibrant health and well-being.

Chapter 2
Understanding Diabetes: Types, Symptoms, and Complications

Before delving into Dr. Barbara's approach to treating diabetes, it's essential to gain a comprehensive understanding of this complex condition. In this chapter, we will explore the different types of diabetes, their symptoms, and potential complications. By understanding the underlying mechanisms of diabetes, we can better appreciate Dr. Barbara's holistic approach to managing the disease and promoting overall health.

Diabetes is a complex metabolic disorder characterized by elevated blood sugar levels resulting from either insufficient insulin production, ineffective insulin utilization, or a combination of both factors. It is a chronic condition that requires careful management to prevent complications and promote overall health and well-being. In this chapter, we will delve into the various types of diabetes, their symptoms, and potential complications.

Types of Diabetes

Type 1 Diabetes: Type 1 diabetes, also known as insulin-dependent diabetes mellitus (IDDM), is an autoimmune condition in which the immune system attacks and destroys the insulin-producing beta cells in the pancreas. This results in little to no insulin production, leading to high blood sugar levels. Type 1 diabetes typically develops during childhood or adolescence but can occur at any age.

Type 2 Diabetes: Type 2 diabetes, formerly known as non-insulin-dependent diabetes mellitus (NIDDM), is the most common form of diabetes, accounting for the majority of cases worldwide. It is characterized by insulin resistance, in which the body's cells become less responsive to insulin, combined with inadequate insulin production. Type 2 diabetes is often associated with lifestyle factors such as obesity, sedentary behavior, and poor dietary habits.

Gestational Diabetes: Gestational diabetes occurs during pregnancy and is characterized by high blood sugar levels that develop or are first recognized during pregnancy. It usually resolves after childbirth, but women who have had gestational diabetes are at increased risk of developing type 2 diabetes later in life.

Symptoms of Diabetes

The symptoms of diabetes can vary depending on the type and severity of the condition but may include:

Frequent urination

Increased thirst

Extreme hunger

Unexplained weight loss

Fatigue

Blurred vision

Slow wound healing

Recurrent infections, such as urinary tract infections or skin infections

Complications of Diabetes

Untreated or poorly managed diabetes can lead to a range of complications that affect various organs and systems in the body. Some common complications of diabetes include:

Cardiovascular Complications: Diabetes significantly increases the risk of cardiovascular diseases such as heart attack, stroke, and peripheral artery disease. High blood sugar levels can damage blood vessels and nerves, leading to atherosclerosis and impaired circulation.

Neuropathy: Diabetes can cause nerve damage (neuropathy) throughout the body, resulting in symptoms such as numbness, tingling, pain, and weakness, particularly in the hands and feet. Diabetic neuropathy can also affect the digestive system, causing gastroparesis (delayed stomach emptying) and other gastrointestinal problems.

Nephropathy: Diabetes is a leading cause of kidney disease (nephropathy), characterized by damage to the kidneys' filtering units (glomeruli). Over time, untreated nephropathy can progress to chronic kidney disease (CKD) and eventually end-stage renal disease (ESRD), requiring dialysis or kidney transplantation.

Retinopathy: Diabetes can damage the blood vessels in the retina (the light-sensitive tissue at the back of the eye), leading to diabetic retinopathy. This condition can cause vision loss or blindness if left untreated.

Foot Complications: Diabetes increases the risk of foot problems such as neuropathy, poor circulation, and foot ulcers. Left untreated, foot ulcers can become infected and may require amputation in severe cases.

Chapter 3
The Role of Nutrition in Diabetes Management

Nutrition plays a crucial role in managing diabetes, influencing blood sugar levels, insulin sensitivity, and overall health. Dr. Barbara emphasizes the importance of a balanced and nutrient-rich diet in supporting individuals with diabetes. In this chapter, we will explore Dr. Barbara's dietary recommendations, including foods to incorporate and avoid, meal planning strategies, and the benefits of adopting a plant-based approach to nutrition.

Nutrition plays a pivotal role in the management of diabetes, influencing blood sugar levels, insulin sensitivity, and overall health outcomes. A well-balanced diet tailored to individual needs can help individuals with diabetes achieve better glycemic control, prevent complications, and improve overall quality of life. In this chapter, we will explore the key principles of nutrition in diabetes management, including dietary recommendations, meal planning strategies, and the importance of adopting a healthy eating pattern.

Carbohydrate Management: Carbohydrates have the most significant impact on blood sugar levels, making carbohydrate management a cornerstone of diabetes nutrition therapy. Individuals with diabetes are encouraged to monitor their carbohydrate intake and choose carbohydrates that have a minimal impact on blood sugar levels, such as whole grains, legumes, fruits, and vegetables. Portion control and carbohydrate counting can help individuals with diabetes manage their blood sugar levels effectively.

Fiber-Rich Foods: Fiber is an essential nutrient for individuals with diabetes as it helps slow down the absorption of sugar in the bloodstream, promoting better blood sugar control. High-fiber foods such as fruits, vegetables, whole grains, legumes, and nuts should be incorporated into the diet regularly to support glycemic control and improve digestive health.

Healthy Fats: Healthy fats play a crucial role in diabetes

management by improving insulin sensitivity, promoting satiety, and supporting heart health. Monounsaturated and polyunsaturated fats found in foods such as avocados, nuts, seeds, olive oil, and fatty fish are preferred choices. Limiting saturated and trans fats from processed and fried foods is essential to reduce the risk of cardiovascular complications.

Protein Sources: Protein is essential for building and repairing tissues and can help stabilize blood sugar levels when consumed as part of a balanced meal. Lean protein sources such as poultry, fish, tofu, legumes, and low-fat dairy products should be included in the diet to promote satiety and support muscle health.

Meal Timing and Distribution: The timing and distribution of meals and snacks throughout the day can impact blood sugar levels and insulin requirements. Eating regular, balanced meals spaced evenly throughout the day can help prevent blood sugar fluctuations and provide sustained energy levels. Consistency in meal timing and portion sizes is key to achieving stable blood sugar control.

Individualized Meal Planning: Diabetes nutrition therapy should be individualized to meet each person's unique needs, preferences, and lifestyle factors. Working with a registered dietitian or certified diabetes educator can help individuals with diabetes develop personalized meal plans that align with their dietary goals, cultural preferences, and medical considerations.

Hydration: Adequate hydration is essential for individuals with diabetes to support kidney function, maintain electrolyte balance, and regulate blood sugar levels. Water is the preferred beverage choice, but unsweetened herbal teas, infused water, and sugar-free beverages can also contribute to overall hydration.

Monitoring and Adjustments: Regular monitoring of blood sugar levels, along with ongoing evaluation of dietary intake and lifestyle habits, is crucial for diabetes management. Making necessary adjustments to the meal plan based on blood sugar readings, medication changes, physical activity levels, and other factors can help individuals with diabetes achieve optimal glycemic control and prevent complications.

Chapter 4
Herbal Remedies and Natural Supplements for Diabetes

In addition to dietary modifications, Dr. Barbara advocates for the use of herbal remedies and natural supplements to support diabetes management. From bitter melon and cinnamon to fenugreek and ginseng, certain herbs and supplements have shown promise in improving blood sugar control and insulin sensitivity. In this chapter, we will explore Dr. Barbara's recommendations for herbal remedies and supplements to complement a holistic approach to diabetes care.

In addition to dietary modifications and lifestyle interventions, herbal remedies and natural supplements can be valuable adjuncts in the management of diabetes. Several herbs and supplements have shown promise in improving blood sugar control, enhancing insulin sensitivity, and supporting overall health in individuals with diabetes. In this chapter, we will explore some of the most commonly used herbal remedies and natural supplements for diabetes management.

Cinnamon: Cinnamon is a popular spice with potent antioxidant and anti-inflammatory properties. Several studies have suggested that cinnamon may help improve insulin sensitivity and lower blood sugar levels in individuals with diabetes. Adding cinnamon to foods and beverages or taking cinnamon supplements may help enhance blood sugar control.

Bitter Melon: Bitter melon, also known as bitter gourd or Momordica charantia, is a tropical fruit that has been used traditionally in Ayurvedic and Chinese medicine to manage diabetes. Bitter melon contains compounds that mimic the action of insulin and may help lower blood sugar levels. Consuming bitter melon as a vegetable or juicing bitter melon fruits may offer potential benefits for individuals with diabetes.

Fenugreek: Fenugreek is an herb commonly used in Indian cuisine and traditional medicine. It contains soluble fiber and compounds that may help improve insulin sensitivity and lower blood sugar levels. Fenugreek seeds can be consumed whole, ground into a powder, or brewed into tea to support diabetes management.

Ginseng: Ginseng is a popular herb used in traditional Chinese medicine for its adaptogenic and anti-diabetic properties. Several studies have shown that ginseng may help improve insulin sensitivity, reduce fasting blood sugar levels, and enhance glycemic control in individuals with diabetes. Ginseng supplements are available in various forms, including capsules, extracts, and teas.

Berberine: Berberine is a compound found in several plants, including goldenseal, Oregon grape, and barberry. Research suggests that berberine may help lower blood sugar levels by increasing insulin sensitivity and reducing insulin resistance. Berberine supplements are available in capsule form and may be beneficial for individuals with diabetes.

Alpha-Lipoic Acid (ALA): Alpha-lipoic acid is a powerful antioxidant that has been studied for its potential benefits in diabetes management. ALA may help improve insulin sensitivity, reduce oxidative stress, and protect against diabetic neuropathy. ALA supplements are available in capsule or tablet form and may be used as part of a comprehensive approach to diabetes care.

Chromium: Chromium is a trace mineral that plays a role in glucose metabolism and insulin signaling. Some studies have suggested that chromium supplementation may help improve insulin sensitivity and lower blood sugar levels in individuals with diabetes. Chromium supplements are available in various forms, including chromium picolinate and chromium chloride.

Aloe Vera: Aloe vera is a succulent plant with anti-inflammatory and anti-diabetic properties. Drinking aloe vera juice or taking aloe vera supplements may help lower blood sugar levels and improve insulin sensitivity in individuals with diabetes. However, more research is needed to fully understand the effects of aloe vera on diabetes management.

Chapter 5
Lifestyle Modifications for Diabetes Prevention and Management

Beyond diet and supplementation, lifestyle modifications are essential for preventing and managing diabetes effectively. Dr. Barbara emphasizes the importance of regular exercise, stress management, adequate sleep, and maintaining a healthy weight in diabetes care. In this chapter, we will explore Dr. Barbara's recommendations for incorporating these lifestyle modifications into daily routines to support overall health and well-being.

Lifestyle modifications are fundamental components of diabetes prevention and management, playing a crucial role in improving blood sugar control, reducing insulin resistance, and lowering the risk of complications associated with diabetes. By adopting healthy habits and making positive changes to diet, physical activity, stress management, and other lifestyle factors, individuals with diabetes can significantly improve their quality of life and overall health outcomes. In this chapter, we will explore key lifestyle modifications for diabetes prevention and management.

Healthy Eating Habits: Adopting a balanced and nutritious diet is essential for diabetes prevention and management. Focus on consuming a variety of nutrient-dense foods, including fruits, vegetables, whole grains, lean protein sources, and healthy fats. Limit intake of processed foods, sugary beverages, refined carbohydrates, and foods high in saturated and trans fats. Portion control and mindful eating practices can help regulate blood sugar levels and support weight management.

Regular Physical Activity: Engaging in regular physical activity is vital for diabetes prevention and management. Aim for at least 150 minutes of moderate-intensity aerobic exercise or 75 minutes of vigorous-intensity aerobic exercise per week, along with muscle-strengthening activities on two or more days per week. Physical activity helps lower blood sugar levels, improve insulin sensitivity, promote weight loss, and reduce the risk of cardiovascular complications associated with diabetes.

Weight Management: Maintaining a healthy weight is essential for diabetes prevention and management. Even modest weight loss can significantly improve blood sugar control and reduce the risk of developing type 2 diabetes. Focus on achieving a healthy body weight through a combination of dietary changes, regular physical activity, and behavior modification strategies. Set realistic goals and monitor progress over time to sustain long-term weight management success.

Stress Reduction Techniques: Chronic stress can contribute to insulin resistance and worsen blood sugar control in individuals with diabetes. Incorporating stress reduction techniques such as mindfulness meditation, deep breathing exercises, yoga, tai chi, and progressive muscle relaxation into daily routines can help lower stress levels and improve overall well-being. Prioritize self-care activities and find healthy ways to cope with stressors to support diabetes management.

Adequate Sleep: Getting adequate sleep is essential for diabetes prevention and management. Poor sleep quality and insufficient sleep duration have been associated with an increased risk of type 2 diabetes and impaired blood sugar control. Aim for seven to nine hours of quality sleep per night and establish a regular sleep schedule to promote optimal sleep hygiene and support overall health.

Limit Alcohol Consumption: Excessive alcohol consumption can interfere with blood sugar control and contribute to weight gain, particularly in individuals with diabetes. Limit alcohol intake to moderate amounts (up to one drink per day for women and up to two drinks per day for men) and avoid binge drinking to minimize the risk of adverse effects on diabetes management and overall health.

Regular Monitoring and Medical Care: Regular monitoring of blood sugar levels, along with routine medical care and follow-up appointments, are essential for diabetes management. Work closely with healthcare providers to develop a personalized treatment plan, set achievable goals, and track progress over time. Be proactive in managing diabetes and communicate any changes in symptoms or concerns with your healthcare team to ensure timely interventions and optimal health outcomes.

Chapter 6
Integrating Dr. Barbara's Approach into Diabetes Care

In the final chapter, we will explore practical strategies for integrating Dr. Barbara's holistic approach into conventional diabetes care. From collaborating with healthcare providers to implementing personalized treatment plans, there are numerous ways to incorporate Dr. Barbara's principles into diabetes management. By embracing a holistic approach that addresses the physical, emotional, and spiritual aspects of health, individuals with diabetes can achieve optimal well-being and thrive in their journey towards health and vitality.

Dr. Barbara's holistic approach to diabetes care offers a comprehensive and personalized approach that emphasizes treating the root causes of the condition, promoting overall well-being, and empowering individuals to take an active role in their health journey.

By integrating Dr. Barbara's principles into diabetes care, healthcare providers can offer a more holistic and patient-centered approach that addresses the physical, emotional, and spiritual aspects of health. In this chapter, we will explore practical strategies for integrating Dr. Barbara's approach into diabetes care.

Comprehensive Assessment: Begin by conducting a comprehensive assessment of the individual's health history, lifestyle habits, dietary patterns, medication regimen, and psychosocial factors. Take a holistic approach to understanding the underlying factors contributing to diabetes and any related complications, including genetic predisposition, environmental influences, and emotional stressors.

Individualized Treatment Plan: Develop an individualized treatment plan tailored to the individual's unique needs, preferences, and goals. Collaborate with the individual to set realistic and achievable goals for blood sugar control, weight management, dietary changes, physical activity, stress management, and other lifestyle modifications. Consider incorporating Dr. Barbara's principles, such as dietary recommendations, herbal remedies, and mind-body practices, into the treatment plan as appropriate.

Nutrition Counseling: Offer nutrition counseling and education to help individuals with diabetes make informed decisions about their dietary choices and meal planning. Emphasize the importance of a balanced diet rich in whole foods, fruits, vegetables, lean protein sources, and healthy fats, while minimizing processed foods, refined carbohydrates, and added sugars. Incorporate Dr. Barbara's dietary recommendations, such as emphasizing plant-based foods, whole grains, and natural sweeteners, into the meal plan.

Herbal Remedies and Supplements: Consider incorporating herbal remedies and natural supplements into the treatment plan to support blood sugar control, improve insulin sensitivity, and promote overall health. Work with individuals to identify safe and effective herbal remedies and supplements that complement conventional diabetes care and align with Dr. Barbara's principles. Monitor the individual's response to herbal remedies and supplements and adjust the treatment plan as needed based on their progress and preferences.

Physical Activity Prescription: Prescribe a personalized exercise program tailored to the individual's fitness level, preferences, and health goals. Encourage regular physical activity, including aerobic exercise, strength training, flexibility exercises, and balance training, to improve blood sugar control, promote weight loss, and reduce the risk of cardiovascular complications. Incorporate Dr. Barbara's emphasis on the importance of regular movement and physical activity in diabetes management.

Stress Management Strategies: Teach stress management techniques and coping strategies to help individuals with diabetes manage the emotional and psychological challenges associated with the condition.

Encourage mindfulness meditation, deep breathing exercises, relaxation techniques, and other mind-body practices to reduce stress levels, improve emotional well-being, and enhance overall quality of life. Integrate Dr. Barbara's holistic approach to stress management into the treatment plan to support individuals in finding balance and resilience amidst the demands of diabetes care.

Regular Monitoring and Follow-Up: Schedule regular monitoring and follow-up appointments to assess the individual's progress, adjust treatment goals and strategies as needed, and provide ongoing support and encouragement. Use objective measures, such as blood sugar levels, weight, blood pressure, and medication adherence, to track the individual's response to treatment and identify areas for improvement. Foster open communication and collaboration between the individual and healthcare team to ensure continuity of care and optimize health outcomes.